Mohamed Jlidi
Walid Bouaicha
Selim Daas

Surgical treatment of isolated capitellum fractures

Mohamed Jlidi
Walid Bouaicha
Selim Daas

Surgical treatment of isolated capitellum fractures

Clinical and radiological functional assessment

ScienciaScripts

Imprint

Any brand names and product names mentioned in this book are subject to trademark, brand or patent protection and are trademarks or registered trademarks of their respective holders. The use of brand names, product names, common names, trade names, product descriptions etc. even without a particular marking in this work is in no way to be construed to mean that such names may be regarded as unrestricted in respect of trademark and brand protection legislation and could thus be used by anyone.

Cover image: www.ingimage.com

This book is a translation from the original published under ISBN 978-620-6-71597-9.

Publisher:
Sciencia Scripts
is a trademark of
Dodo Books Indian Ocean Ltd. and OmniScriptum S.R.L publishing group

120 High Road, East Finchley, London, N2 9ED, United Kingdom
Str. Armeneasca 28/1, office 1, Chisinau MD-2012, Republic of Moldova, Europe
Printed at: see last page
ISBN: 978-620-7-89759-9

INTRODUCTION

Capitellum fractures are rare. They account for less than 1% of all elbow fractures. This is a partial frontal lesion of the distal end of the humerus. These injuries can lead to joint callus, post-traumatic osteoarthritis, stiffness, pain and instability. [1]. These coronal shear fractures of the capitellum are the result of axial compression of the capitellum by the radial head [2].

The diagnosis of a capitellum fracture is made using plain radiographs of the elbow, but the extent of the fracture is often underestimated on this initial radiological work-up, while non-displaced or osteochondral lesions may even remain hidden[3,4]. CT scans are generally required for assessment, classification and surgical planning.

Orthopedic treatment has lost its place, as these articular fractures require anatomical reduction and early mobilization.

Surgical treatment has evolved from closed-focus osteosynthesis or simple excision of the fragment to open internal fixation using either cortical screws or direct screws with buried heads. Herbert and Scarf screws have several advantages over cannulated screws. They enable fracture compression with minimal damage to articular cartilage [5]. This allows early rehabilitation and does not require removal of the hardware. Their high cost remains a limitation to their use. The use of either technique remains dependent on surgeons' habits and the availability of technical facilities. Few studies have compared these two therapeutic approaches [6].

The aim of our study is to investigate the functional, clinical and radiological results of surgical treatment of capitellum fractures, and to compare these results according to the means of osteosynthesis.

METHODS

1. Type of study

This is a single-center retrospective study conducted in the orthopedics and traumatology department of Mohamed Tahar Maâmouri Hospital in Nabeul, over a 6-year period from January 2016 to December 2022, focusing on the surgical treatment of capitellum fractures.

2. Study population :

2.1.   Inclusion criteria

We included in our study patients with:

- ❖ Over 18 years of age
- ❖ Isolated capitellum fracture treated surgically
- ❖ A usable file (observation notebook and a complete radiological check-up preoperatively, postoperatively and at final follow-up)
- ❖ Hindsight of over 6 months.

2.2.   Exclusion criteria

We have excluded :

- ❖ Patients lost to follow-up
- ❖ An inoperable case (radiological findings missing preoperatively, postoperatively or at the last follow-up)
- ❖ Associated fracture of the trochlea

2.3.   Non-inclusion criteria

- ❖ Age under 18
- ❖ Other elbow fractures: olecranon, supra- and inter-condylar...
- ❖ Orthopedically treated fractures
- ❖ Less than 6 months
- ❖ Pathological fracture
- ❖ Associated fracture of the humeral shaft or radial head.

3. Methods :

3.1.   Data collection

We consulted the archives of the orthopedic surgery and traumatology department of the Mohamed Taher Maamouri university hospital in Nabeul for the period from January

2016 to December 2022. We collected 31 observations classified as capitellum fracture. After checking the inclusion and exclusion criteria, we retained 22 observations. The clinical and radiological data of each patient were recorded on a previously established form.

3.2.   Epidemiological profile

For each patient we noted:

- ❖ Age at time of trauma
- ❖ The sex
- ❖ Medical and surgical history
- ❖ Habits: smoking
- ❖ Patient origin: urban or rural
- ❖ The dominant side
- ❖ The profession
- ❖ The circumstances in which the trauma occurred

3.3.   Clinical examination

Inspection revealed functional impotence of the upper limb. Mobilization of the elbow aroused pain. Vasculo-nerve complications were systematically investigated.

The complete somatic examination looked for associated abdominal, thoracic, cranial or musculoskeletal lesions.

3.4.   Radiological examination

Standard X-rays were taken systematically, and included a frontal and lateral view of the elbow.

A CT scan is requested to better analyze the fracture and rule out another associated fracture (Figure 1).

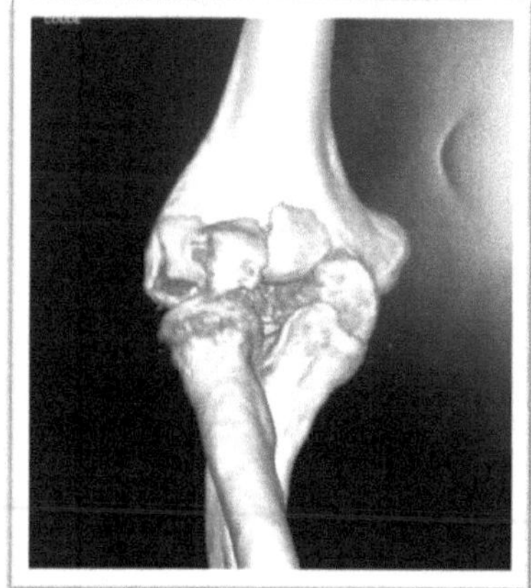 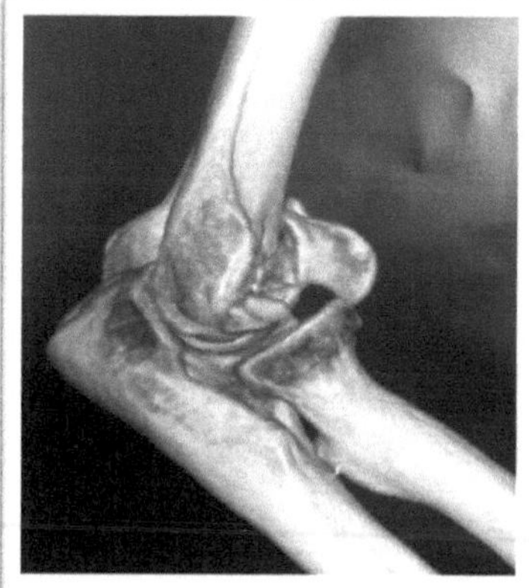

Figure 13D scan sections showing a comminuted fracture of the capitellum

We used the classification of Bryan and Morrey [7,8]. Capitellum fractures are classified into four types (Figure 2):

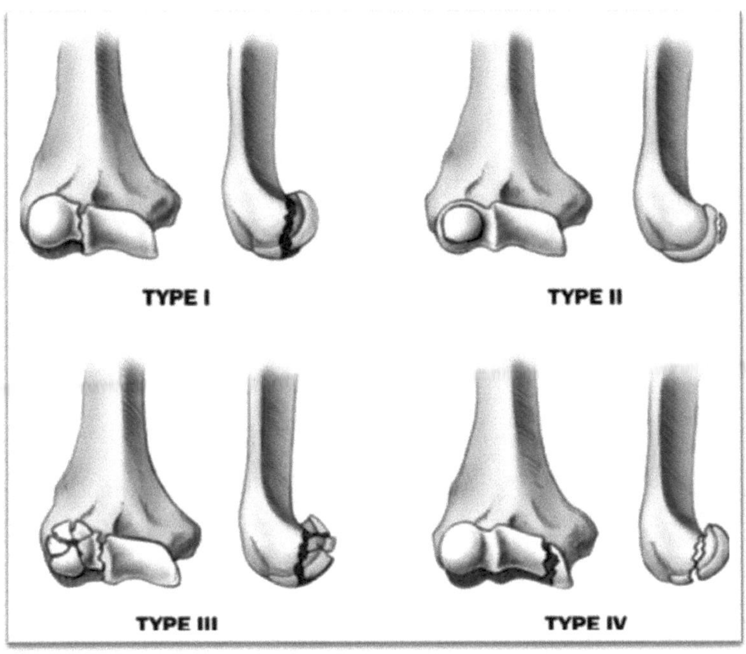

Figure 2 Bryan and Morrey classification

Type I: The Hahn-Steinthal fracture involves a large part of the capitellum. The trochlea is only minimally involved (Figure 3).

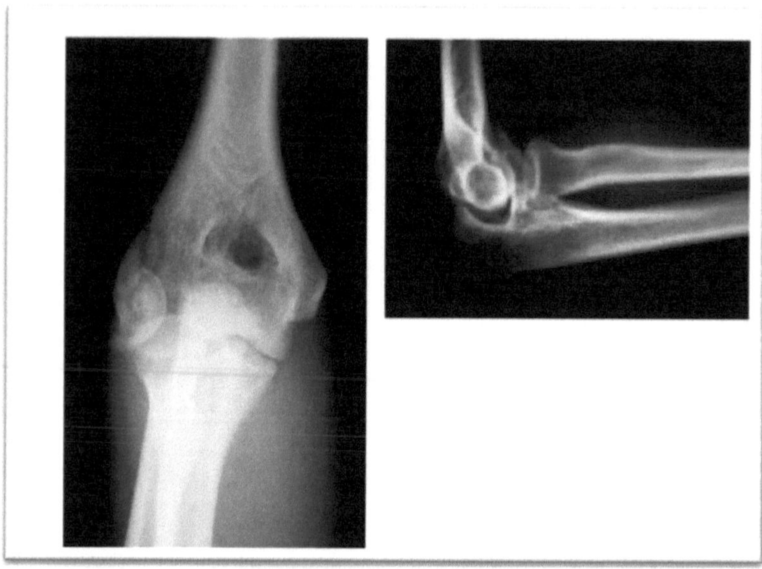

Figure 3 Fracture capitellum type 1

Type II, also known as the Kocher-Lorenz fracture, is a separation fracture of the articular cartilage with very little subchondral bone attached (Figure 4).

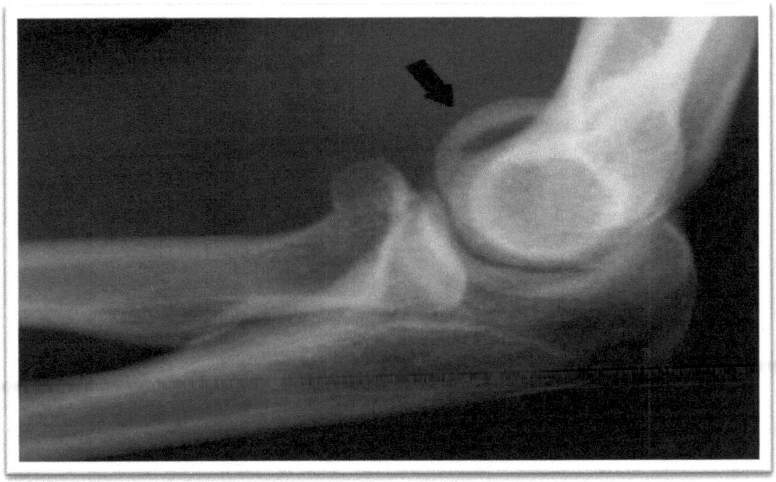

Figure 4 Fracture capitellum type 2

Type III is a multi-fragmentary fracture, as shown in Figure 5.

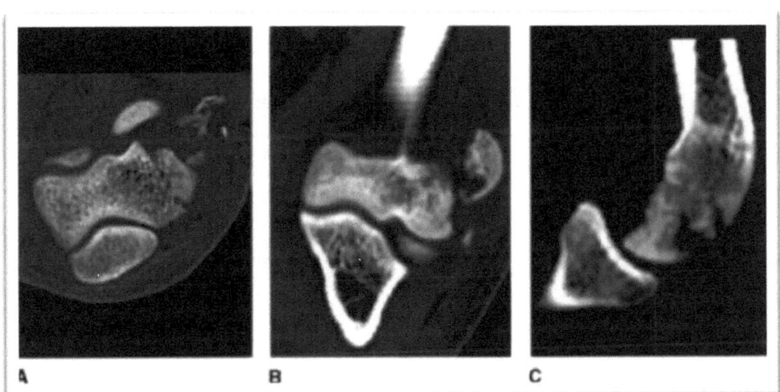

Figure 5capitellum fracture type 3

McKee added a type IV which is a coronal plane fracture involving the capitellum and part of the trochlea as a single segment (Figure 6).

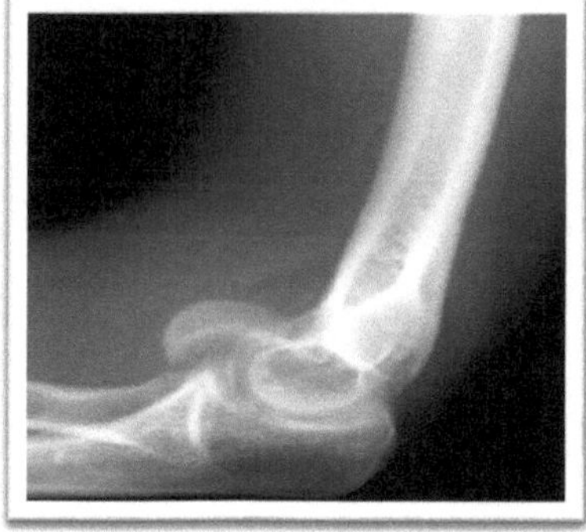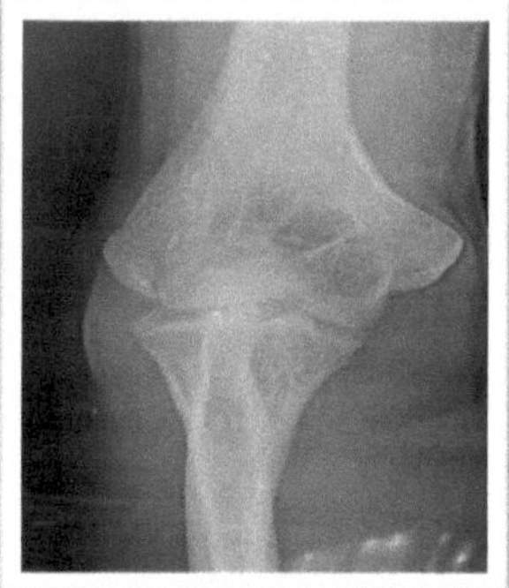

Figure 6 Fracture capitellum type 4

3.5. Surgical treatment

3.5.1. Operating time

Delay in treatment is defined by the time between the trauma and the surgical procedure.

3.5.2. Type of anesthesia

The procedure is performed either under general anesthesia or locoregional anesthesia.

3.5.3. Type of osteosynthesis devices

Two types of implants were used in our series:

3.5.3.1. Scarf screws

Scarf screws are buried-head screws that allow direct screwing into the capitellum (Figure 7).

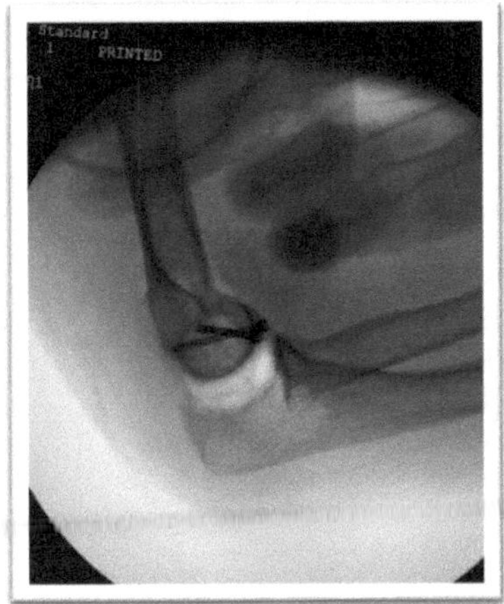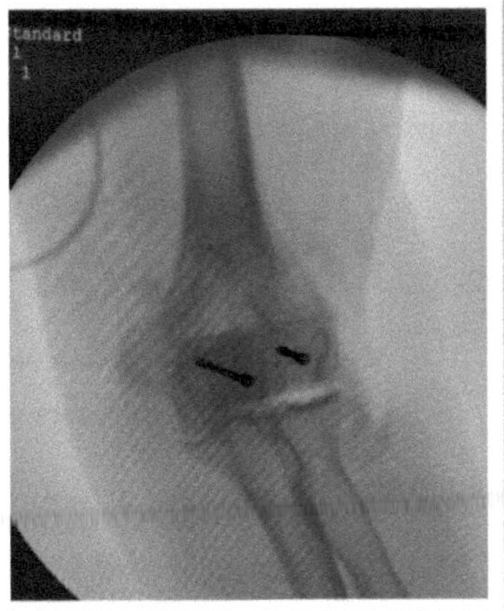

Figure 7 Osteosynthesis **of** a capitellum fracture using direct screw fixation with a scarf screw

3.5.3.2. Cortical screws

Stabilization of the capitellum fracture can be achieved with a posteroanterior screw-retraction technique using one or two cortical screws (Figure 8). [9,10].

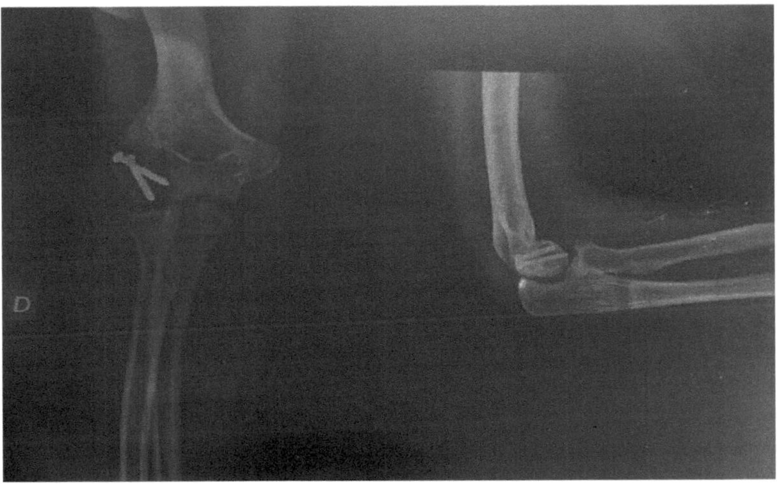

Figure 8 Osteosynthesis of capitellum fracture using two retaining screws

11

3.5.4. Approach

All patients underwent surgery via an external elbow approach.

3.5.5. Length of hospital stay

The number of days from hospitalization to discharge.

3.6.   Post-operative follow-up
3.6.1. Post-operative care

Prophylactic antibiotic therapy for 48 hours and analgesics were instituted.

3.6.2. Immobilization

All patients were immobilized with a brachio- ante brachial splint.

3.6.3. Rehabilitation

Rehabilitation was systematically indicated. Its aim was to prevent stiffness and amyotrophy.

4. Evaluation of results
4.1.   Functional and clinical assessment
4.1.1. Visual analog scale :

Pain was assessed by VAS for all patients [11].

4.1.2. Elbow mobility

We evaluated :

- ❖ The extension
- ❖ Bending
- ❖ Pronation
- ❖ Supination

4.1.3. Mayo elbow performance score

The Mayo elbow performance score [12] is a self-administered questionnaire. It is designed to assess elbow mobility limitations due to pathology, in daily life; its maximum score is 100. It uses 4 sub-scores: pain, mobility, stability and daily gestures involving the elbow (Appendix 1).

4.1.4. American Shoulder and Elbow Score (ASES)

The American Shoulder and Elbow Score (ASES) [13,14] is a reliable and valid tool for assessing shoulder and elbow function [5]. The ASES has also been standardized for the assessment of elbow function, with a patient self-assessment section and a physician assessment section. (Appendix 2)

4.2. Radiological assessment

Standard radiographs were used to assess fracture consolidation, to identify any secondary displacement or debricolage of the osteosynthesis material, and to monitor the development of complications.

4.3. Complications

4.3.1. Aigues

❖ Infection
❖ Volkman syndrome
❖ Other

4.3.2. Chronicles

❖ Algodystrophy
❖ Pseudarthrosis
❖ Elbow stiffness and ankylosis
❖ Vicious callus (figure 9)

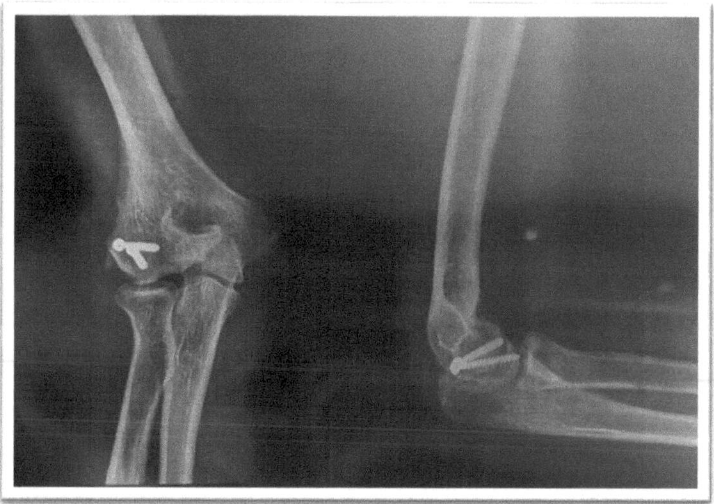

Figure 9: Cal vicieux of a capitellum fracture

* Osteoarthritis of the elbow
* Instability
* Periarticular ossification
* Unscrambling equipment
* Intra-articular material protrusion (figure 10)

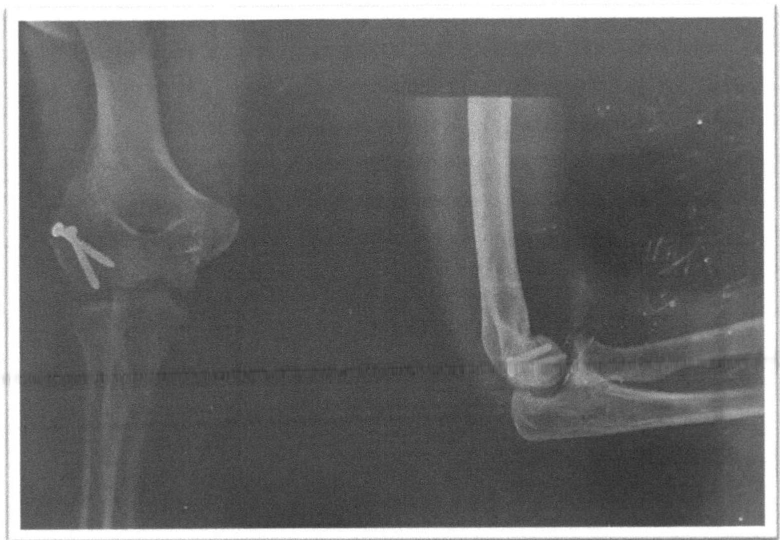

Figure 9 Intra-articular material protrusion

5. Statistical analysis

Data were entered using SPSS software version 26.0.

Statistical analysis was performed using SPSS software version 26.0.

We calculated absolute frequencies and relative frequencies (percentages) for qualitative variables. We calculated means, medians and standard deviations and determined extreme values for quantitative variables.

Comparisons of means on independent series were made using the Mann Whitney U test. Comparisons of percentages on independent series were made using Pearson's chi-square test, and in the event of significance in the chi-square test and non-validity of this test and comparison of two percentages, by Fisher's two-tailed exact test.

6. Bibliographic research

We carried out a bibliographic search, analyzed theses and studied trauma-orthopedics books available at the four Tunisian medical faculties, in order to discuss and compare our results with data in the literature. The bibliographic search was carried out on the Pub Med portal with the following keywords: Fracture du capitellum (capitellar fracture), osteosynthesis (ostheosynthesis), surgical treatment (surgery) and complications (complication). The articles were subsequently downloaded from Science Direct, EM Premium and Springer Link. Some articles were freely available on journal sites (AJR, Joint Bone J Surg Br...).

7. Ethics and patient consent

All patients included in this work were informed that their data would remain confidential, and that consultation was authorized only by those collaborating on this work. No patient refused. No conflicts of interest are to be declared.

RESULTS

1. Epidemiological parameters :

1.1. Age :

The mean age of our patients was 42.77 ± 42.77 years, with extremes ranging from 21 to 68 years. The distribution of patients by age group is illustrated in figure 11.

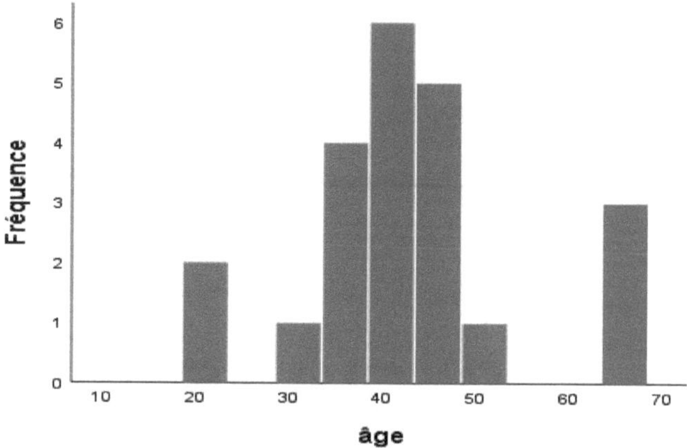

Figure 11: Patient distribution by age group

1.2. Genre:

In this series, there was a clear predominance of females, with a sex ratio of 0.57 (figure 12).

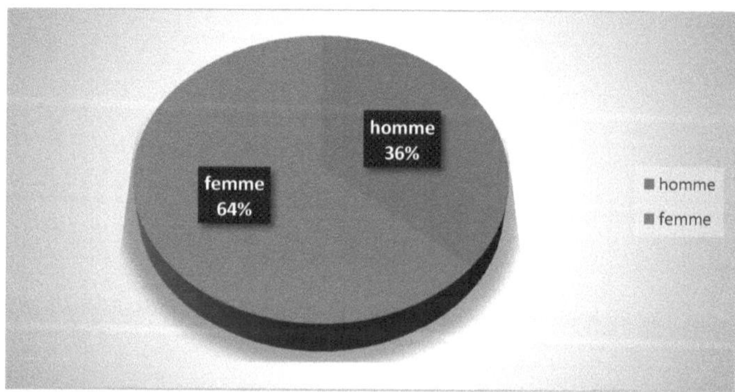

Figure 10 Patient distribution by gender

1.3. Profession:

Sedentary workers and patients with no work were predominant (86% of cases) (figure 13).

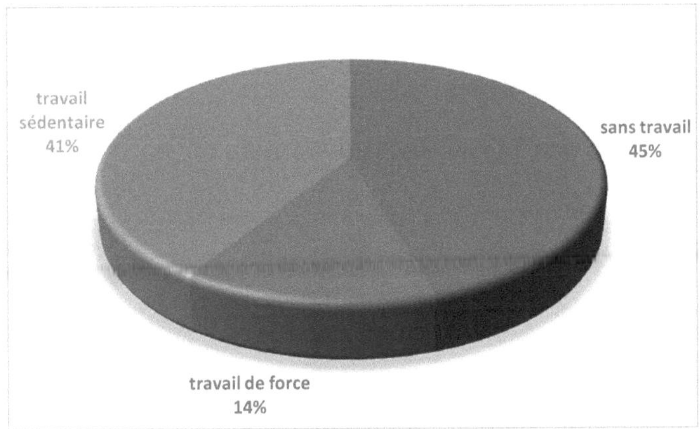

Figure 11 Distribution of patients by profession

1.4. History and comorbidities:

The majority of patients (55%) had no significant pathological history. Diabetes predominated (18%) (Table I).

Table I Distribution of patients by history

	Number	%
ATCD	10	45%
Diabetes	4	18%
Cardiovascular history	3	14%
Other	5	23%

1.5. Smoking :

Five patients were active smokers. All smokers were men.

1.6. Origin:

We noted that 73% of patients lived in rural areas (N=16 cases) versus 25% in urban areas (N=6 cases).

2. Clinical study:

2.1. Reached:

The right elbow was the most affected (60%). No bilateral involvement was noted in our series. The side was dominant in 19 cases (86%).

2.2. Mechanism:

Domestic accidents were the most frequent (69%) (figure 14).

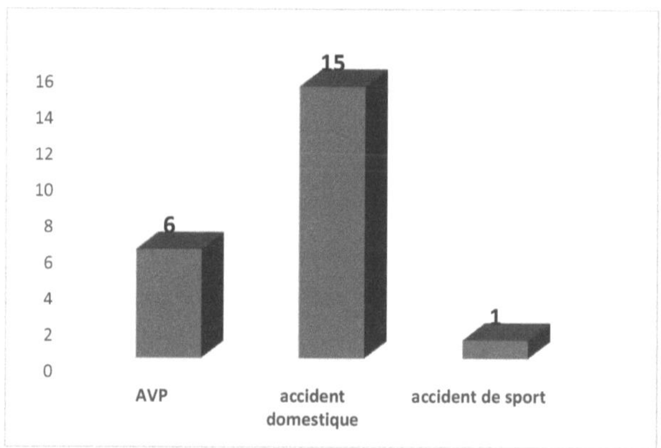

Figure 12 Distribution of patients by circumstances of trauma

3. Physical examination :

Pain was the most common symptom (91%). No skin openings or vascular-nerve complications were reported (Table II).

Table II Distribution of symptoms

Factor	Workforce	Percentage
Pain	20	91%
total functional impotence	10	45%
Elbow deformity	3	14%
Oedema	1	5%

4. Radiological study

All our patients underwent radiography of the elbow from the front and side. CT scans were requested in 11 cases (50%). The majority of fractures were classified as type I (45%) according to the modified Brayn and Morrey classification (figure 15).

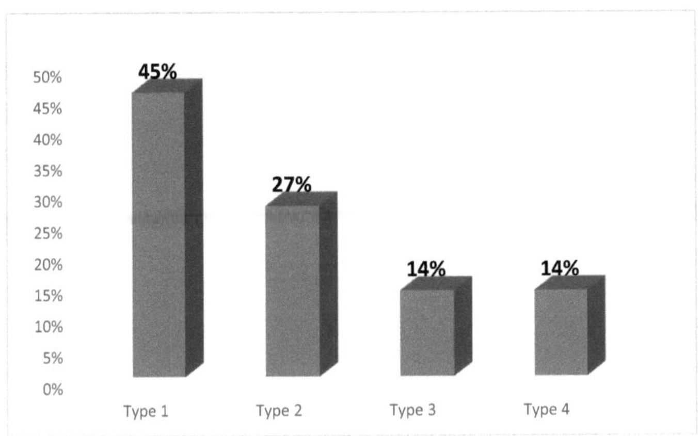

Figure 13 Distribution of fractures according to the modified Brayn et Morrey classification

5. Therapeutic management:

5.1. type of anesthesia

63.63% of patients underwent general anaesthesia.

5.2. Operating time :

The average operating time was 3.9 days, with extremes ranging from 1 to 7 days.

5.3. Approach :

The external anterolateral elbow approach was used for all patients.

5.4. Type of osteosynthesis:

The most common type of material used was 3.5 cortical screws (76% of cases) (figure 16).

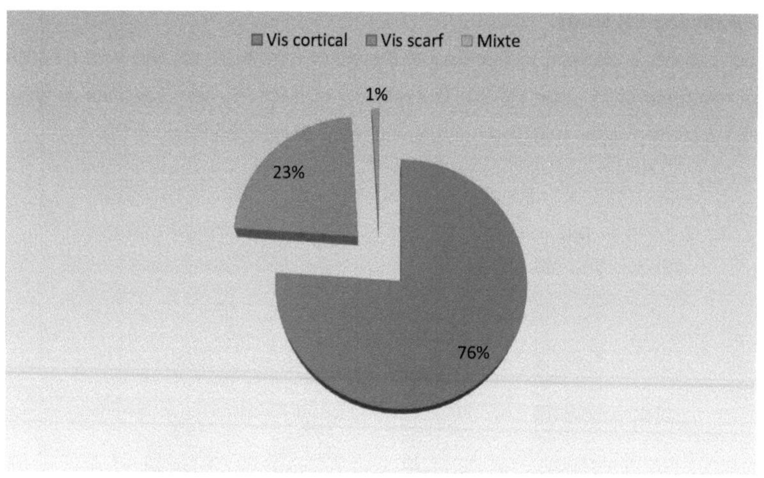

Figure 14 Distribution of patients by osteosynthesis method

Four fractures were stabilized by direct screw fixation. Posterior-anterior screw fixation was used in 17 cases. These two techniques were used together in only one case.

5.5.　Length of stay :

The average hospital stay was 5.77 days, with extremes ranging from four to seven days.

6.　Postoperative follow-up:

6.1.　Postoperative treatment :

Analgesic treatment and antibiotic prophylaxis were prescribed for all patients.

6.2.　Downtime:

The average length of immobilization was 21 days, with extremes ranging from 16 to 26 days.

6.3.　Rehabilitation

Rehabilitation was prescribed for all patients. The average number of sessions was 39.14, with extremes ranging from 25 to 54 sessions.

7. Late secondary complications:

7.1. Acute complication

No acute complications were noted.

7.2. Chronic complication

Algodystrophy was reported in two patients. Elbow stiffness was noted in four cases. Vicious callus was found in only one patient.

Three patients developed post-traumatic osteoarthritis. Intra-articular material protrusion was noted in only one case.

8. Functional results:

The mean follow-up was 25.36 months, with extremes ranging from 12 months to 72 months.

8.1. Pain :

The mean VAS score was 1.9 [1 - 3].

8.2. Elbow mobility:

At last recoil, patients had a mean flexion of 137.5°. Joint amplitudes are shown in Table III.

Table III Joint amplitudes at last recoil

	Average	Median	Minimum	Maximum
Bending (°)	137,5	140	90	150
Extension (°)	-19,77	-20	-55	0
Pronation (°)	74,32	80	45	90
Supination (°)	56,82	65	0	90

8.3. Back to work :

All patients who performed sedentary work returned to work within an average of 10 weeks. In the case of patients performing strenuous work, only three did not return to work.

8.4. ASES score

The mean ASES score was 72.32, ranging from 64 to 80.

8.5. Mayo elbow performance score

The mean Mayo Clinic elbow performance index was 90.2 (Table IV).

Table IV Distribution according to Mayo Clinic index

	MEPS	Pain	Mobility	Stability	Function
Average	90,2	41,8	16,8	10	21,6
Minimum	85	40	15	10	20
Maximum	100	45	20	10	25
Median	85	40	15	10	20

9. Radiological result

The fracture was consolidated in all patients within an average of 45 days. Delayed consolidation was noted in three cases.

10. Functional results by technique :

We divided our population according to the means of osteosynthesis into :

- ❖ Group A: includes 17 fractures stabilized by screw-retraction using 3.5 cortical screws.
- ❖ Group B: includes four patients treated with direct screwing using Scarf screws

10.1. Pain :

The mean VAS score was 2 in both techniques, with no significant difference (p=0.27).

10.2. Elbow mobility:

At final recoil, Group B patients had better flexion, but with no significant difference (p=0.085) (Table V).

Table V Repair of flexion measurement according to osteosynthesis method

Means of osteosynthesis	Average	Minimum	Maximum	P
Scarf	145	135	150	0,085
Screw 3.5	135,29	90	150	

Patients in group A had a mean extension of -26 compared with a mean extension of -18 for patients in group B. (p=0.218) (Table VI)

Table VI Repair of extension measurement according to osteosynthesis method

	Average	Minimum	Maximum	P
Scarf	-26	-40	-15	0,218
Screw 3.5	-17,94	-55	0	

There was no significant difference in the mean pronation value between the two groups (p=0.493) (Table VII).

Table VII Repair of pronation measurement according to osteosynthesis method

	Average	Minimum	Maximum	P
Scarf	71	55	90	0,493
Screw 3.5	75,29	45	90	

For supination, we noted that the average in group A was greater but with no significant difference (p=0.058) (Table VIII).

Table VIII Repair of supination measurement by osteosynthesis method

	Average	Minimum	Maximum	P
Scarf	43	20	55	0,058
Screw 3.5	60,88	0	90	

10.3. ASES score

The osteosynthesis technique had no significant influence on the ASES score (Table IX)

.

Table IX Repair of supination measurement according to osteosynthesis method

ASES	Average	Minimum	Maximum	P
Scarf	71,4	64	80	0,543
Screw 3.5	72,59	70	80	

10.4. Mayo Clinic Performance Index

Mean Mayo Clinic performance index measurements were higher in patients in group B. This difference was significant (p=0.038) (Table X).

Table X Repair of Mayo Clinic performance index averages by osteosynthesis method

	Scarf		Screw 3.5		P
	Average	Median	Average	Median	
MEPS	96	100	89	85	0,038

Pain	44,00	45,00	41,18	40,00	0,020
Mobility	19,00	20,00	16,18	15,00	0,020
Stability	10,00	10,00	10,00	10,00	
Function	23,00	25,00	21,18	20,00	0,136

10.5. Chronic complications according to osteosynthesis type

The rate of chronic complications was higher when the SCARF screw was used, but not significantly so (Table XI).

Table XI Repair of chronic complications by type of osteosynthesis

	Scarf		Screw 3.5		P
	Number	%	Number	%	
algodystrophy	1	20%	1	6%	0,358
Stiffness	0	0%	4	24%	0,251
Vicious callus	0	0%	1	6%	0,6
Osteoarthritis	2	40%	4	24%	0,491
Material projection	1	20%	0	0%	0,063

DISCUSSION

Capitellum fractures are rare, with an estimated prevalence of between 0.5 and 1% of all adult elbow fractures [15]. Orthopedic treatment is becoming increasingly obsolete, as these articular fractures require anatomical reduction and early mobilization. [3]. Surgical treatment has evolved from closed-focus osteosynthesis or simple excision of the fragment to open internal fixation using either cannulated or direct cannulated screws. Herbert and Scarf screws have several advantages over cannulated screws [10]. They enable fracture compression with minimal damage to articular cartilage. This enables early rehabilitation and does not require removal of the hardware. Their high cost remains a limitation to their use. The use of either technique remains dependent on surgeons' habits and the availability of technical facilities. Few studies have compared these two therapeutic approaches.

We conducted a monocentric retrospective study in the traumatology-orthopedics department of the Mohamed Tahar-Maâmouri Nabeul University Hospital, over a period of 6 years, on the surgical treatment of capitellum fractures.

The aim of our study was to investigate the functional, clinical and radiological results of surgical treatment of capitellum fractures, depending on the osteosynthesis method used.

1.   Epidemiological profile

1.1.   Age and gender

The mean age in our series was 42.77 ± 42.77 years, with extremes ranging from 21 to 68 years, and this is consistent with the literature. Indeed, the mean age of adults presenting with capitellum fracture varies between 37.5 and 63 years according to studies [16-20].

In a series of type IV capitellum fractures, the mean age of patients with capitellum fractures was 32 years. [17]. In contrast, Najib A et al. [18] found that the majority of patients with capitellum fractures were over 75 years of age, and that women were more affected by these fractures than men.

Author	Year	Workforce	Average age (years)
Tanriverdi et al.	2020	16	40
Kapil Mani KC et al.	2020	21	39
Fang et al.	2023	5	54,6
Yoshida et al	2021	16	49
Our Series	2023	22	44,7

Table XII: Variation in age according to the literature

According to the literature, the gender distribution of patients with capitellum fractures varied from study to study. Pavić R et al [21] found a predominance of females in his series of 35 patients with isolated capitellum fractures, with a sex ratio of 0.75. These results are consistent with our series, in fact, the sex ration in our study is 0.57.

In a series of 101 cases, Ha C et al. [22] studied capitellum fractures associated with fractures of the head or neck of the radius. He reported that concomitant capitellum fractures occur more frequently in women.

However, we found many series with a male predominance. Indeed, Rausch V et al [16] found a sex ratio of 2.1. Furthermore, a review of 14 cases treated by open reduction and internal fixation with Herbert screws revealed that nine patients were male and five female [15]Schmidt et al. found that these fractures occur most frequently in young men or elderly women. [20].

These epidemiological variations can be explained by patient selection.

Author	Year	Workforce	Percentage

			Male/Female
Cheungsoo Ha	2023	101	53,5/46,5
Pavic R	2012	35	42,8/57,2
Our series	2023	22	36/64

Table XIII: Gender variations in the literature

1.2. Affected side and dominant side

In our series, the right elbow was most affected (60%). Our results are consistent with the series by Singh et al, who found that the side most affected was the right side in patients with type IV capitellum fractures [23]. However, Cheungsoo et al.[24] noted that the most affected side was the left.

In the study by Wolfson et al, published in Clinical Orthopaedics and Related Research, conducted on 100 patients with capitellum fractures, found that 64% of fractures involved the dominant side[25]. Similarly, Szabo TG et al, in a series including 150 patients with capitellum fractures, found that 67% of fractures involved the dominant side [26]. In our study, the dominant side was involved in 86% of fractures. Involvement of the dominant side may have a greater functional impact, especially in manual and heavy-duty workers.

1.3. Comorbidity

In our series, the majority of patients had no notable pathological history. Returning to the literature, the incidence of comorbidities is variable, with a higher prevalence in older patients [27]. However, in these elderly subjects, the biomechanical stability of simple coronal shear fractures of the capitellum is not significantly affected by these comorbidities [28]. In the case of displaced fractures, headless compression screw fixation can provide stable fixation, with good to excellent functional results [29].

Another study reported that distal humerus fractures, which may include capitellum fractures, are associated with comorbidities such as hypertension, diabetes and obesity [30,31]. In addition, a review of 14 cases of capitellum fractures treated by open reduction and internal fixation with Herbert screws reported that only one patient had a history of rheumatoid arthritis [17]. Therefore, although there is no clear evidence of specific comorbidities common in capitellum fractures, it is important to consider the potential complications associated with these fractures, such as avascular necrosis and elbow instability in elderly patients with tarsias.

1.4. Mechanism

The most common mechanism of capitellum fractures is a fall onto the palm of the hand with the elbow in extension [32]. These fractures are most often the result of high-energy trauma. Road accidents were the most frequent cause, accounting for 62.5% of cases [33]. In our series, the most frequent mechanism was a domestic accident (69% of cases). Our results are not in line with the literature, and this may be explained by the small sample size.

Other mechanisms have been reported, such as direct trauma to the elbow.

2. Clinical examination

The reason for consultation varies. Elbow pain, swelling, deformity and functional impotence are the most commonly described in the literature. [11]. Elbow deformity is most obvious in cases of associated dislocation. The diagnosis of a fracture of the head or neck of the radius can also be a reason for discovering an associated capitellum fracture [1].

3. Classifications

There are several classification systems for capitellum fractures, including the modified classification of Bryan and Morrey [7]Hume's classification [6]Dubberley's classification [1] and Jupiter's classification [7]
The most commonly used classification is that of Bryan and Morrey. It comprises four types of fracture, depending on the extent of the fracture:

> ❖ Type I (Hahn-Steinthal fracture): complete osteochondral fracture of the capitellum; the trochlea may also be involved.

- ❖ Type II (Kocher-Lorenz fracture): anterior osteochondral shear fracture with minimal subchondral bone involvement.
- ❖ Type III (Broberg-Morrey fracture): compressed or comminuted fracture of the capitellum.
- ❖ Type IV: Coronal shear fracture involving the capitellum and extending to the trochlea

Several classifications have been developed, but their reliability and accuracy have been called into question [3,34]. Currently, various research studies suggest that a more comprehensive classification system should take into account the type of these three-dimensional fractures, the displacement of the different fragments and the impact of the on treatment results [35].

In our study, all patients underwent radiographic examination of the elbow from the front and in profile. The majority of fractures (45%) were classified as type I according to the modified Brayn et Maurey classification. In the literature, and comparable to our results, **Yu et al**. reported in a series of 26 patients that type I capitellum fractures are the most frequent (48% of cases) [65]. These findings were validated by **Garner et al** [66] with a percentage of 75% of type I fractures, and by Trinh et al. where type I accounted for 84% of capitellum fractures in a meta-analysis including 28 studies [67].

3. **Radiological examination :**

The initial radiological work-up includes a strict frontal and lateral X-ray, which in most cases confirms the diagnosis. In the case of displaced fractures, the pathognomonic sign of McKee's double arch is often visible on a profile X-ray, where the two arches visible separately represent the displaced capitellum and the trochlea. The extent of capitellum fractures is often underestimated on this radiological assessment. Moreover, non-displaced lesions may remain hidden. Computed tomography is generally indispensable for assessment, classification and surgical planning [36].

4. **Therapeutic management**

Treatment of a capitellum fracture depends on the type of fracture. Some authors propose orthopedic treatment for non-displaced or slightly displaced fractures in elderly subjects with reduced functional demand or who are not anaesthetizable [37]. However, for most authors, surgery remains the mainstay of treatment for these fractures [38]. Open reduction is indicated in all displaced capitellum fractures and in those in which closed reduction fails. Anatomical reduction, stable fixation and early mobilization of the elbow joint are important for optimal results [3].

Several therapeutic modalities have been described:

- ❖ Surgical excision: the presence of significant comminution may prevent fixation; surgical excision of fragmented fragments is then recommended [10].
- ❖ Screw fixation: Open reduction and internal fixation (ORIF) is the most commonly used technique for treating capitellum fractures. Various implants are described in the literature.

Indeed, Wolfson et al [25] described the technique of osteosynthesis of capitellum fractures using compression screws with buried heads. For improved biomechanical stability, Sen et al. [39] recommended the use of anti-slip plates combined with compression screws. In our series, the most commonly used technique is cortical screws. With the development of the medical industry, screws with recessed heads are increasingly used.

The most commonly reported approach in the literature is an external elbow approach, which offers a good view of the fracture and control of reduction. For small joint fragments, Ring et al. [40] recommend an extended lateral approach.

5. Functional and clinical evaluation :
5.1. Pain
5.1.1. Pain assessment

The VAS is a common and simple method for assessing post-operative pain. It is a scale graduated from 0 to 10, where 0 represents the absence of pain and 10 represents the most intense pain imaginable. VAS can be used to assess pain before and after surgical treatment, as well as to monitor pain during post-operative rehabilitation [41]. In our series, the mean VAS was 1.9 [1-3], in line with the observations of authors such as Roujdi et al [58] and Kaufmann et al [59].

5.1.2. Functional and clinical scores
a. ASES score

American Shoulder and Elbow Surgeons Score (ASES) [13] is a questionnaire developed to assess shoulder and elbow function. The score is a 100-point scale composed of two parameters: pain and activities of daily living. The pain score is worth 50 points and the activities of daily living score is worth 50 points. The pain and activities of daily living scores are then added together to obtain the final ASES score (out of 100) [13]. This score is widely used in the English-speaking world. Indeed, in a systematic review of the literature, Flynn et al. observed that the ASES is the third most widely used score (16% of studies) for assessing the long-term results of capitellum fractures treated with any technique [61].

In our study, the mean ASES score was 72.32, ranging from 64 to 80. Our results are comparable with the literature. Indeed, in a prospective study by **Guitton et al.** including 88 partial capitellum fractures, the mean ASES score was 88 points [42]. In another study by Hech Z et al. including 15 patients with capitellum fractures treated with fine-threaded Kirschner wires, the mean ASES score was 91.5 [43].

b. The Mayo Elbow Performance Index (MEPI):

The Mayo Elbow Performance Index (MEPI) is a scoring system used to assess functional outcomes in patients with elbow fractures, including capitellum fractures. The score is divided into four categories: pain, range of motion, stability and function. The score ranges from 0 to 100, with higher scores indicating better outcomes.[44].

The mean MEPI score in our series was 90.2, in line with most studies. In the series by Singh et al, involving 14 cases of displaced capitellum I fractures treated by ORIF with Herbert screws, the mean score was 89.3. Eight patients had excellent results and three had good results [17]. Yoshida et al. in their series of 26 capitellum fractures, found that nine patients had excellent results (MEPI≥ 90), nine had good results (75 ≤MEPI≤89) and eight had fair results (60≤MEPI≤74) [45].

Bienvenu et al. described three cases of capitellum fractures treated by ORIF with Herbert screws with buried heads.[46]. Functional assessment according to the MEPI score was considered excellent for all three patients, with scores of 94, 96 and 98. Similarly, the mean MEPI score for the 20 patients was 92.5 in the series by Sultan et al. [47].

5.2. Joint amplitudes :

In our series, mean elbow flexion was 137.5°. Mean extension was -19.77°. Mean pronosupination was 74.32° and 56.82° respectively. Our results were consistent with most series.

Returning to the literature, Singh (2009) reports positive results in 14 cases treated with Herbert screws, with all patients achieving a stable, pain-free elbow and good joint amplitude [17,23]. Open reduction and internal fixation, with the aim of achieving a stable anatomical reduction and early rehabilitation, is a guarantee of a better functional outcome.

Several studies [15,17] have noted a loss of elbow mobility, in particular limited extension and/or flexion, after surgical treatment of capitellum fractures. The degree of loss of mobility depends on the severity of the fracture, the treatment used and post-operative rehabilitation.

Indeed, capitellum fractures are known to limit elbow range of motion. Post-traumatic stiffness is observed in up to 40% of patients, even with early mobilization after open reduction and internal fixation. Despite this stiffness, several authors have reported good to excellent results [48-50].

In the series by Hulet et al. [51] of capitellum fractures treated with ORIF, the mean elbow motion angles at last follow-up were 4° extension (0-30), 138° flexion (130-145), 83° supination and 83° pronation.

Belmoubarek et al. reported the case of a neglected capitellum fracture in a 36-year-old woman with limited functional needs [15]. On initial examination, flexion was limited to 95° with free extension and pronosupination. After surgical reduction of the callus and osteosynthesis by anteroposterior screw fixation in compression with a single countersunk screw, pain had disappeared and mobility was satisfactory with flexion at 130°, extension at 0°, pronation at 90° and supination at 90° [15].

In another descriptive study by Mani K C et al. including 22 capitellum fractures treated by ORIF using Herbert screws, the mean movements for pronation and supination were 161.59 ± 6.79 degrees respectively at a mean setback of 37.45 ± 9.43 weeks (28-58 weeks) [22].

In the same context, Bienvenu et al. described three observations of capitellum fractures treated by direct screw fixation using Herbert screws. Joint amplitudes were restored at 3 months post-operatively [52].

In addition, Ogawa et al. presented a case of a patient with excision of a capitellum fracture fragment. He found that pronosupination was complete [52].

Kotte et al. and Zwerus et al. reported statistically significant correlations between elbow flexion-extension and pronosupination. They found that functional outcome is not affected by a slight decrease in joint amplitudes [53,54].

5.3. Resuming work :

Resumption of work and daily activity after a capitellum fracture varies in the literature, depending on the type of fracture and the therapeutic method used. In our study, all patients who performed sedentary work returned to work within an average of 10 weeks. In the case of patients who performed strenuous work, only three did not return to work. Returning to the literature, return to work depends essentially on the quality of the reduction, the primary stability of the fixation and the rehabilitation programme [51,55]. D. Andrew Hulet et al studied the return to work of capitellum fractures treated by ORIF with Herbert screws. Of the 14 patients who had been working at the time of the accident, 13 had returned to work at the last follow-up. This return-to-work rate was high in all occupational categories, including manual workers, office workers and professionals. This author stresses the importance of rehabilitation and especially its early start [51].

6.   Radiological evaluation :

In our series, the average consolidation time was 45 days. Delayed consolidation was observed in only three cases. Our results are comparable to those reported by Ruchelsman et al. who reported a mean consolidation time of 50 days in his series of 16 patients treated with ORIF [67]. HC et al. noted that the mean time to consolidation was 4.2 months [19].

The duration of consolidation in capitellum fractures may vary depending on the anatomopathological type of fracture, the comminution and the treatment method used. Kapil Mani K C et al [56]. in a series of 22 capitellum fractures treated by ORIF with

Herbert screws, found that the mean duration of consolidation was 11.13±1.20 weeks (9-15). This is longer than our study.

7. Complications:

7.1. Acute complications :

In our study, we reported no acute complications. Our results are consistent with most series in which acute complications such as sepsis are very rare. [6,57].

7.2. Chronic complications :

Chronic complications of capitellum fractures are common. In our series, the most frequent chronic complication was elbow stiffness (18.18% of cases). Returning to the literature, in a recent meta-analysis including 42 studies, The most reported complications after surgical fixation of capitellum fractures included elbow pain (21%), radiocapitellar arthritis (19%), hardware removal (17%) and heterotopic ossifications (13%) [57].

Elbow stiffness is a widespread complication, irrespective of the surgical method used. Indeed, in a meta-analysis of capitellum fractures treated by excision, the most reported complication was elbow stiffness[58].

In our series, other complications are similar to those reported in this meta-analysis. Indeed, post-traumatic osteoarthritis was noted in 13.63% of cases. These results are similar to those found by Baydar et al. [59]. This author noted a post-traumatic osteoarthritis rate of 14.28%. In contrast, Dubberley et al. [60] found a higher rate of post-traumatic osteoarthritis (32.14% of cases). This high rate is explained by the frequency of post-traumatic cartilage lesions of the capitellum discovered intraoperatively.

In our study, all fractures were consolidated. Returning to the literature, the rate of pseudarthrosis varies between 0 and 30%. [58]. In a recent study by Nagashree et al. involving 61 patients, the pseudarthrosis rate was 8.19%. [61]. This complication is more frequently reported in comminuted fractures and fractures of the capitellum with extension to the trochlea.

The rates of heterotopic ossifications vary in the literature [58] However, in most studies, the quantity of ossifications is not determined. These ossifications do not have a significant functional impact and do not require surgical treatment [62]. In our series, heterotopic ossifications did not occur. This may be explained by the small sample size.

The frequency of avascular necrosis is expected to be high in capitellum fractures, as the fragment is avascular with little soft tissue attachment. However, avascular necrosis of the capitellum has been reported to be very rare in several studies [58]. The prevalence of this complication may be related to the severity of the initial injury, including posterior comminution. In many studies, the majority of cases were observed in the Ring classification of type 3 or higher [63]. In our series, the occurrence of this complication was not noted.

The last reported complication is post-traumatic osteoarthritis. In a meta-analysis including 42 articles, radiocapital osteoarthritis was reported in 19% of cases. [57]. In contrast, Nagashree et al.[61] noted a lower rate of osteoarthritis (3.27%). This may be explained by the small sample size and short follow-up time. In our series, the rate of osteoarthritis is higher, estimated at 27.27% of cases. This rate is higher in elderly subjects.

8. Results by osteosynthesis method

In our series, we found better results for patients treated with anteroposterior screw fixation. Pain was significantly reduced for both techniques, with a mean VAS of 2. Concerning elbow mobility, at last recoil, patients treated with anteroposterior screw fixation using Scarf screws had better joint mobility in the sagittal plane, with no significant difference. For pronosupination, joint amplitudes were better in the group of patients treated with Scarf screws, but the difference was not statistically significant. The ASES score was slightly higher in patients treated with posterior-anterior screws, but the difference was not significant (p=0.54). Whereas, patients treated with Scarf screws had better MEPI scores than those treated with 3.5 cortical screws, with a statistically significant difference (p=0.03).

Returning to the literature, the functional and clinical results of capitellum fractures treated with ORIF are variable. In a descriptive cross-sectional study including 22 patients by KC KM et al. fixation of the capitellum fracture with a Herbert screw resulted in rapid recovery of elbow function, with a mean Mayo score of 91.5 [56]. These results are consistent with observations reported by Makhni et al [14] and Singh et al [20].

Hulet et al. in a series of 14 cases of capitellum fractures with or without trochlear extension treated by ORIF using Herbert screws, reported a mean extension of 4°, a mean flexion of 138°, a mean supination of 83° and a mean pronation of 83° [51].

As regards capitellum fractures treated with posterior-anterior screw fixation, the studies are long-standing. Dubberley et al.[60] in a series of 11 cases, studied the functional and clinical results of patients treated with 3.5 cortical recall screws. The mean Mayo score was (91 ± 11). Mean elbow mobility ranged from 19° to 138°. Widhalm et al. in a series of 13 patients treated with posterior-anterior screw fixation, found a mean ASES score of 37.8 and a mean Mayo score of 92.7. Mean flexion was 138.8° ± 7.6° [120-150°] and mean extension deficit was 4.9° ± 10.4° [-25 to 10°]. Mean pronation was 88.8° ± 4.0° [80-95°] and mean supination was 85.8° ± 7.3° [70-90°][64].

Our results are close to these series.

As regards complications, in our series we found no significant difference between the two fixation methods. Returning to the literature, a recent meta-analysis of 42 studies compared the two groups according to the direction of screw fixation. The average rate of avascular necrosis of the capitellum was higher in the posterior-anterior direction (29% versus 11%). The rate of fixation revision (2.9% vs. 6.7%) and heterotopic ossification (7.3% vs. 22%) was higher in the anteroposterior direction. Transient paralysis of the posterior interosseous nerve was reported in four patients in four studies, three of whom had anteroposterior screw fixation[57].

CONCLUSION

Fractures of the capitellum are rare lesions. These coronal shear fractures of the capitellum are the result of axial compression of the capitellum by the radial head. These injuries can lead to joint callus, post-traumatic osteoarthritis, stiffness, pain and instability.

We conducted a monocentric retrospective study conducted at the orthopedics and traumatology department of Mohamed Tahar Maâmouri Hospital in Nabeul, spread over a 6-year period from January 2016 to December 2022, focusing on the surgical treatment of capitellum fractures.

The aim of our work is to study the functional, clinical and radiological results of surgical treatment of capitellum fractures and to compare these results according to the means of osteosynthesis.

We included patients aged over 18 with an isolated capitellum fracture treated surgically with a minimum 6-month follow-up.

We excluded orthopedically-treated capitellum fractures, those under 18 years of age, other elbow fractures (olecranon, supra- and inter-condylar, etc.), associated fractures of the humeral shaft or radial head, and files that could not be processed.

Twenty-two cases were included in our study. The mean age was 50.68 years. The sex ratio was 0.29. Five patients were active smokers. Fractures involved 13 right elbows (60%) and 9 left elbows (40%). Domestic accidents were the most frequent mechanism of injury (69% of cases).
Total functional impotence and pain were the most frequent symptoms.
All our patients underwent radiographic examination of the elbow from the front and in profile. CT scans were performed in 11 patients (50%).
We used the modified Brayn et Maurey classification to classify capitellum fractures. Type I is the most frequent (45% of cases).
The average operating time was 3.9 days. All our patients underwent external elbow surgery. The fracture was fixed by anteroposterior screw fixation using Scarf screws in four cases, and recoil screw fixation using 3.5 screws in 17 cases. Only one case was treated with a combination of these two methods of osteosynthesis. The mean duration of immobilization was 21 days, with extremes ranging from 16 to 26 days. The average hospital stay was 5.77 days.

The mean follow-up was 25.36 months, with extremes ranging from 12 to 72 months. At last recoil, the mean VAS score was 1.9. Mean flexion was 137.5°. Mean extension was -19.77°. Mean pronation was 74.32° and mean supination was 56.82°.

The mean ASES score was 72.32 and the mean Mayo Clinic Performance Index measure was 90.2.

The fracture was consolidated in all patients within an average of 45 days. However, delayed consolidation was noted in 4 cases.

No acute complications were noted in our series.

As regards chronic complications, algodystrophy was reported by 2 patients, elbow stiffness was noted in 4 cases, and a callus was found in one patient. Six patients developed post-traumatic osteoarthritis, and a protrusion was noted in only one case.

Comparing the two means of osteosynthesis, the mean VAS score was 2 for both techniques. The osteosynthesis technique had no significant influence on the ASES score. Mean Mayo Clinic performance index measurements were higher in the Scarf technique, with a statically significant difference (p=0.038).

Patients using a 3.5 screw had a mean flexion of 135°, compared with 145° when the Scarf technique was used (p=0.078). The use of a 3.5 screw was associated with a mean extension of -26°, compared with -18° when Scarf screws were used (p=0.197). There was no significant difference in mean pronation between the two techniques (p=0.477). For supination, we noted that the mean value in the group of patients treated with 3.5 screws was greater, but the difference was not statistically significant (p=0.053).

In terms of chronic complications, we noted 40% algodystrophy, 40% osteoarthritis and 20% protrusion in patients treated with direct screw fixation using Scarf screws. In patients treated with 3.5 screws, we noted 24% stiffness and 24% osteoarthritis. No significant differences were found.

In conclusion, our study and the results reported in the literature suggest that both types of osteosynthesis offer distinct advantages, each with its own specific features and indications. De Scarf screw fixation seems to offer stability and precise reduction in certain cases of isolated capitellum fracture, while 3.5 screws have the advantage of low cost and fewer chronic complications.

REFERENCES

1.   Suresh S. Type 4 capitellum fractures: Diagnosis and treatment strategies. Indian J Orthop. 2009;43(3):286-91.

2.   Garner M, Schottel P, Hotchkiss R, Daluiski A, Lorich D. Capitellum Fracture Fragment Excision: a Case Series. HSS J. August 1, 2015;11.

3.   Picart B, Ferreira A, Malherbe M. Functional management of a type II capitellum fracture in a female volleyball player. J Traumatol Sport. March 1, 2021;38(1):37-9.

4.   Tajika T, Hatori Y, Kuboi T, Saida R, Chikuda H. Articular shear fracture of the capitellum in a child: A case report. JOS Case Rep [Internet]. 25 Nov 2023 [cited 27 Nov 2023]; Available from: https://www.sciencedirect.com/science/article/pii/S2772964823000576

5.   Yang W, Tian T, Wu HY, Pan QJ, Dang S, Sun ZM. Syntheses and structures of a series of uranyl phosphonates and sulfonates: an insight into their correlations and discrepancies. Inorg Chem. 2013 March 4;52(5):2736-43.

6.   Hu SK, Xu L, Guo JH, Liao JP, Qin TW, Huang FG. The impact of associated injuries and fracture classifications on the treatment of capitellum and trochlea fractures: A systematic review and meta-analysis. Int J Surg Lond Engl. June 2018;54(Pt A):37-47.

7.   McKee MD, Jupiter JB, Bamberger HB. Coronal shear fractures of the distal end of the humerus. J Bone Joint Surg Am. Jan 1996;78(1):49-54.

8.   Tanwar YS, Kharbanda Y, Jaiswal A, Birla V, Pandit R. Retrospective analysis of open reduction and internal fixation of coronal plane fractures of the capitellum and trochlea using the anterolateral approach. SICOT-J. 4:8.

9.   Mighell MA, Harkins D, Klein D, Schneider S, Frankle M. Technique for internal fixation of capitellum and lateral trochlea fractures. J Orthop Trauma. 2006;20(10):699-704.

10.   BAYDAR M, AYKUT S, MERT M, KESKINBIÇKI MV, AKDENIZ HE, ÖZTÜRK K. ISOLATED CAPITELLAR FRACTURE FIXATION WITH HEADLESS SCREWS IN DIFFERENT CONFIGURATIONS. Acta Ortop Bras. 30(1):e244357.

11.   Rosas S, Paço M, Lemos C, Pinho T. Comparison between the Visual Analogue Scale and the Digital Assessment Scale in the perception of aesthetics and pain. Int Orthod [Internet]. Dec 1, 2017 [cited Jan 9, 2024];15(4):543-60. Available from: https://www.sciencedirect.com/science/article/pii/S1761722717301225

12.   Stanborough RO, Bestic JM, Peterson JJ. Shoulder Osteoarthritis. Radiol Clin North Am. Jul 2022;60(4):593-603.

13.   Agel J, Hebert-Davies J, Braman JP. American Shoulder and Elbow Surgeons score: what does it tell us about patients selecting operative treatment of a rotator cuff injury? JSES Int. Sept 2023;7(5):751-5.

14.   Makhni EC, Saltzman BM, Meyer MA, Moutzouros V, Cole BJ, Romeo AA, et al. Outcomes After Shoulder and Elbow Injury in Baseball Players: Are We Reporting What Matters? Am J Sports Med. Feb 2017;45(2):495-500.

15.   Belmoubarik A, Achargui A, Azagui Y, Bennouna D. Neglected capitellum fracture in an adult: about a case and review of the literature. Pan Afr Med J. Feb 27, 2015;20:184.

16.   Rausch V, Königshausen M, Schildhauer TA, Gessmann J, Seybold D. Fractures of the capitellum humeri and their associated injuries. Obere Extrem. 2018;13(1):33-7.

17.   Singh AP, Singh AP, Vaishya R, Jain A, Gulati D. Fractures of capitellum: a review of 14 cases treated by open reduction and internal fixation with Herbert screws. Int Orthop. August 2010;34(6):897-901.

18.   Najib A, Rifi M, Moustain MR, Berrada MS, Yaacoubi ME. SURGICAL TREATMENT OF CAPITELLUM FRACTURES IN ADULTS. 2012;

19.   Ha C, Lee JK, Kim S, Jo S, Chung J, Han SH. Incidence and typology of concomitant capitellum fractures associated with radial neck and radial head fractures. Rev Chir Orthopédique Traumatol. 1 Sep 2023;109(5):692-3.

20.   Chamseddine A, Hamdan H, Obeid B, Zein H. Frontal articular fractures of the distal end of the humerus. Chir Main. 2009 Dec 1;28(6):352-62.

21.   Pavić R, Malović M. Isolated capitellum humeri fractures in adults. Coll Antropol. march 2012;36(1):187-94.

22.   Ha C, Lee JK, Kim S, Jo S, Chung J, Han SH. Incidence and pattern of concurrent capitellum fracture associated with radial head and neck fractures. Orthop Traumatol Surg Res OTSR. Sept 2023;109(5):103531.

23.   Singh AP, Dhammi IK, Garg V, Singh AP, Shuang-ming S. Outcome of surgical treatment of type IV capitellum fractures in adults. Chin J Traumatol. August 1, 2012;15(4):201-5.

24.   Cheung EV. Fractures of the capitellum. Hand Clin. nov 2007;23(4):481-6, vii.

25.   Wolfson TS, Lowe D, Egol KA. Capitellum fracture open reduction and internal fixation with headless screws. J Orthop Trauma. August 2019;33 Suppl 1:S5-6.

26.   Szabo TG, Simovitch M, Hak DJ, Altchek DA. Fractures of the capitellum: a review of 150 cases. J Orthop Trauma. 2012;26(9):587-92.

27.   Lopiz Y, Rodríguez-González A, García-Fernández C, Marco F. Open reduction and internal fixation of coronal fractures of the capitellum in patients older than 65 years. J Shoulder Elbow Surg. March 2016;25(3):369-75.

28.   Borbas P, Vetter M, Loucas R, Hofstede S, Wieser K, Ernstbrunner L. Biomechanical stability of simple coronal shear fracture fixation of the capitellum. J Shoulder Elbow Surg. August 2021;30(8):1768-73.

29.   Mighell M, Virani NA, Shannon R, Echols EL, Badman BL, Keating CJ. Large coronal shear fractures of the capitellum and trochlea treated with headless compression screws. J Shoulder Elbow Surg. Jan 2010;19(1):38-45.

30.   Moayeri A, Mohamadpour M, Mousavi SF, Shirzadpour E, Mohamadpour S, Amraei M. Fracture risk in patients with type 2 diabetes mellitus and possible risk factors: a systematic review and meta-analysis. Ther Clin Risk Manag. 11 Apr 2017;13:455-68.

31.   Werner BC, Rawles RB, Jobe JT, Chhabra AB, Freilich AM. Obesity is associated with increased postoperative complications after operative management of distal humerus fractures. J Shoulder Elbow Surg. oct 2015;24(10):1602-6.

32.   De Boeck H, Pouliart N. Fractures of the capitellum humeri in adolescents. Int Orthop. 2000;24(5):246-8.

33. Paneri DJ, Kala DA, Gupta DS. Capitellum fracture: Outcome of surgical treatment. Int J Orthop Sci. 2020;6(2):656-60.

34. Laulan J, Marteau E, Bacle G. The MEU classification system for fractures of the distal end of the radius. Prognostic and therapeutic interests of an independent analysis of different fracture parameters. Hand Surg Rehabil. Dec 1, 2016;35:S28-33.

35. De Thomasson E, Rouvreau Ph, Begue Th, Leriche de Cheveigne C, Mathoulin Ch, Boury G, et al. Limitations and inadequacies of treatments for recent double-jointed fractures of the lower quarter of the radius. Ann Chir Main Memb Supér. Jan 1, 1994;13(1):13-9.

36. Kunkel S, Cornwall R, Little K, Jain V, Mehlman C, Tamai J. Limitations of the radiocapitellar line for assessment of pediatric elbow radiographs. J Pediatr Orthop. Sept 2011;31(6):628-32.

37. Hachimi K, Hattoma N, Sennoune B, Rafai M, Largab A, Trafeh M. Surgical treatment of capitellum fractures in adults. About eight cases. Chir Main. 1 Apr 2004;23(2):79-84.

38. Tanriverdi B, Kural C, Altun S. Capitellum fractures: Treatment with headless screws and outcomes. Jt Dis Relat Surg. June 18, 2020;31(2):291-7.

39. Sen MK, Sama N, Helfet DL. Open Reduction and Internal Fixation of Coronal Fractures of the Capitellum. J Hand Surg [Internet]. Nov 1, 2007 [cited Feb 15, 2024];32(9):1462-5. Available from: https://www.jhandsurg.org/article/S0363-5023(07)00709-5/abstract

40. Ring D. Open Reduction and Internal Fixation of an Apparent Capitellar Fracture Using an Extended Lateral Exposure. J Hand Surg [Internet]. Apr 1, 2009 [cited Feb 15, 2024];34(4):739-44. Available from: https://www.jhandsurg.org/article/S0363-5023(09)00105-1/abstract

41. Sabatino MJ, Jo CH, Wilson PL, Ellis HB. ARE SELF-REPORTED PAIN SCALES IN PEDIATRICS VALID? Orthop J Sports Med. March 29, 2019;7(3 Suppl):2325967119S00039.

42. Guitton TG, Doornberg JN, Raaymakers ELFB, Ring D, Kloen P. Fractures of the capitellum and trochlea. J Bone Joint Surg Am. Feb 2009;91(2):390-7.

43. Heck S, Zilleken C, Pennig D, Koslowsky TC. Reconstruction of radial capitellar fractures using fine-threaded implants (FFS). Injury [Internet]. feb 2012 [cited May 8, 2024];43(2):164-8. Available from: https://linkinghub.elsevier.com/retrieve/pii/S0020138311001732

44. Stavrakakis IM, Sylignakis P, Magarakis GE, Ntontis Z, Chaniotakis C, Alvanos A. Capitellum and trochlea fractures. A systematic review of the literature. J Clin Orthop Trauma. August 1, 2022;31:101922.

45. Yoshida S, Sakai K, Nakama K, Matsuura M, Okazaki S, Jimbo K, et al. Treatment of Capitellum and Trochlea Fractures Using Headless Compression Screws and a Combination of Dorsolateral Locking Plates. Cureus. 13(3):e13740.

46. Bienvenu BPKP, Amine ER, Khalid C, Mohamed A, Mohamed El, Mohamed S, et al. Hahn Steinthal fracture treated with Herbert screw fixation: 3 cases. Pan Afr Med J. Jan 13, 2015;20:30.

47. Sultan A, Khursheed O, Bhat MR, Kotwal HA, Manzoor QW. Management of capitellar fractures with open reduction and internal fixation using Herbert screws. Ulus Travma Ve Acil Cerrahi Derg Turk J Trauma Emerg Surg TJTES. nov 2017;23(6):507-14.

48. Zhang D, Nazarian A, Rodriguez EK. Post-traumatic elbow stiffness: Pathogenesis and current treatments. Shoulder Elb. Feb 2020;12(1):38-45.

49.   Mahmood B. Management of Post-traumatic Elbow Stiffness. Oper Tech Orthop. March 1, 2023;33(1):101027.

50.   Mittal R. Posttraumatic stiff elbow. Indian J Orthop. 2017;51(1):4-13.

51.   Hulet DA, D'Auria JL, Earp BE, Zhang D, Benavent K, Blazar PE. Long-Term Outcomes and Return to Work After Isolated Coronal Shear Fractures of the Capitellum. J Hand Surg Glob Online. March 10, 2023;5(3):310-4.

52.   Ogawa T, Shirasawa S. Conservative treatment in displaced fractures of the humeral capitellum: a reduction technique under local anaesthesia. BMJ Case Rep. 17 Apr 2018;2018:bcr2017223820.

53.   Kotte SHP, Viveen J, Koenraadt KLM, The B, Eygendaal D. Normative values of isometric elbow strength in healthy adults: a systematic review. Shoulder Elb. Jul 2018;10(3):207-15.

54.   Zwerus EL, Willigenburg NW, Scholtes VA, Somford MP, Eygendaal D, van den Bekerom MP. Normative values and affecting factors for the elbow range of motion. Shoulder Elb. June 2019;11(3):215-24.

55.   Fisher KJ, Livesey MG, Sax OC, Gilotra MN, O'Hara NN, Henn RF, et al. Are outcomes after fixation of distal humerus coronal shear fractures affected by surgical approach? A systematic review and meta-analysis. JSES Int. 13 Sep 2022;6(6):1054-61.

56.   KC KM, Acharya P, Marahatta SB, Sigdel A, KC A, Dahal SC. Functional Outcomes of Capitellum Fractures Treated by Open Reduction and Internal Fixation with Herbert Screw: A Descriptive Cross-sectional Study. JNMA J Nepal Med Assoc. Oct 2020;58(230):775-9.

57.   Heller M, Abdelaal MS, Adams A, Ilyas AM, Kachooei AR. Rate of Complications After Capitellum Fracture Fixation: A Systematic Review and Meta-Analysis. J Hand Surg [Internet]. nov 2023 [cited May 9, 2024];S0363502323005907. Available from: https://linkinghub.elsevier.com/retrieve/pii/S0363502323005907

58.   Carroll MJ, Athwal GS, King GJW, Faber KJ. Capitellar and Trochlear Fractures. Hand Clin [Internet]. nov 2015 [cited May 9, 2024];31(4):615-30. Available from: https://linkinghub.elsevier.com/retrieve/pii/S0749071215000803

59.   BAYDAR M, AYKUT S, MERT M, KESKINBIÇKI MV, AKDENIZ HE, ÖZTÜRK K. ISOLATED CAPITELLAR FRACTURE FIXATION WITH HEADLESS SCREWS IN DIFFERENT CONFIGURATIONS. Acta Ortop Bras [Internet]. 24 Nov 2023 [cited 24 Nov 2023];30(1):e244357. Available from: https://www.ncbi.nlm.nih.gov/pmc/articles/PMC8979352/

60.   Dubberley JH. Outcome After Open Reduction and Internal Fixation of Capitellar and Trochlear Fractures. J Bonė Jt Surg Am [Internet]. Jan 1, 2006 [cited May 9, 2024];88(1):46. Available from: http://jbjs.org/cgi/doi/10.2106/JBJS.D.02954

61.   Nagashree V, Dheenadhayalan J, Sundaram VP, Zackariya M, Sivakumar S, Vembanan K, et al. Outcome determinants for coronal shear fractures of the distal humerus. Int Orthop [Internet]. May 2024 [cited May 11, 2024];48(5):1295-302. Disponible sur: https://link.springer.com/10.1007/s00264-024-06151-2

62.   Bilsel K, Atalar AC, Erdil M, Elmadag M, Sen C, Demirhan M. Coronal plane fractures of the distal humerus involving the capitellum and trochlea treated with open reduction internal fixation. Arch Orthop Trauma Surg [Internet]. 2013 June [cited 2024 May 11];133(6):797-804. Disponible sur: http://link.springer.com/10.1007/s00402-013-1718-5

63. Byun YS, Shin DJ, Dan JM, Lee SM, Jeong DG, Gu TH, et al. Clinical Results of Open Reduction and Internal Fixation in the Coronal Plane Articular Fracture of the Distal Humerus. J Korean Orthop Assoc [Internet]. 2016 [cited May 11, 2024];51(4):301. Available from: https://jkoa.org/DOIx.php?id=10.4055/jkoa.2016.51.4.301

64. Widhalm HK, Seemann R, Wagner FT, Sarahrudi K, Wolf H, Hajdu S, et al. Clinical outcome and osteoarthritic changes after surgical treatment of isolated capitulum humeri fractures with a minimum follow-up of five years. Int Orthop. Dec 2016;40(12):2603-10.

APPENDICES

Table I Mayo Elbow Performance Score[7,9]

	No. of points[*]
Pain (45 points)	
None	45
Mild	30
Moderate	15
Severe	0
Range of motion (20 points)	
>100° flexion arc	20
50°-100° flexion arc	15
<50° flexion arc	5
Stability (10 points)	
Stable	10
Mild instability (<10° of varus-valgus laxity)	5
Gross instability (≥10° of varus-valgus laxity)	0
Daily function (25 points)	
Combing hair	5
Feeding oneself	5
Hygiene	5
Putting on shirt	5
Putting on shoes	5
Maximum possible (total)	100

[*] The outcome is rated as follows: excellent, 90 to 100 points; good, 75 to 89 points; fair, 60 to 74 points; or poor, less than 60 points.

Appendix 1: The Mayo elbow performance score

ASES - Orthopaedic Scores

ASES Shoulder Score

Name .... Age .... Date ....

D

1. Usual Work

2. Usual Sport/Leisure activity?

3. Do you have shoulder pain at night?
- ○ Yes
- ○ No

4) Do you take pain killers such as paracetamol (acetaminophen), diclofenac,
- ○ Yes
- ○ No

5) Do you take strong pain killers such as codeine, tramadol, or morphine?
- ○ Yes
- ○ No

6) How many pills do you take on an average day?

7) Intensity of pain?

○ 10   ○ 9   ○ 8   ○ 7   ○ 6   ○ 5   ○ 4   ○ 3   ○ 2   ○ 1

Pain as bad as it can be

8) Is it difficult for you to put on a coat?
- ○ Unable to do
- ○ Very difficult to do
- ○ Somewhat difficult
- ○ Not difficult

9) Is it difficult for you to sleep on the affected side?
- ○ Unable to do
- ○ Very difficult to do
- ○ Somewhat difficult
- ○ Not difficult

10) Is it difficult for you to wash your backside up bra?
- ○ Unable to do
- ○ Very difficult to do
- ○ Somewhat difficult
- ○ Not difficult

11) Is it difficult for you manage toiletting?
- ○ Unable to do
- ○ Very difficult to do
- ○ Somewhat difficult
- ○ Not difficult

12) Is it difficult for you to comb your hair?
- ○ Unable to do
- ○ Very difficult to do
- ○ Somewhat difficult
- ○ Not difficult

13) Is it difficult for you to reach a high shelf?
- ○ Unable to do
- ○ Very difficult to do
- ○ Somewhat difficult
- ○ Not difficult

14) Is it difficult for you to lift 10lbs. (4.5kg) above your shoulder?
- ○ Unable to do
- ○ Very difficult to do
- ○ Somewhat difficult
- ○ Not difficult

15) Is it difficult for you to throw a ball overhand?
- ○ Unable to do
- ○ Very difficult to do
- ○ Somewhat difficult
- ○ Not difficult

16) Is it difficult for you to do your usual work?
- ○ Unable to do
- ○ Very difficult to do
- ○ Somewhat difficult
- ○ Not difficult

17) Is it difficult for you to do your usual sport/leisure activity?
- ○ Unable to do
- ○ Very difficult to do
- ○ Somewhat difficult
- ○ Not difficult

The Total ASES score is: 0

18: This page cannot be saved due to patient data protection so please print the filled in form before closing the window

Page design : Aaron Rooney

Reference : American Shoulder and Elbow Surgeons Standardized Shoulder Assessment Form p
section reliability, validity, and responsiveness Michener LA, McClure PW, Sennett BJ J Shoulder E
Nov-D

Appendix 2: The American Shoulder and Elbow Score (ASES)

Table of contents

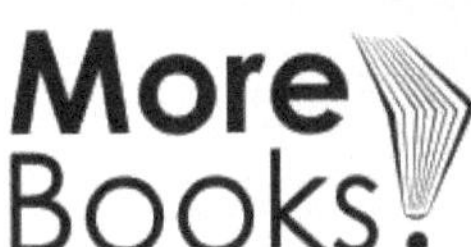

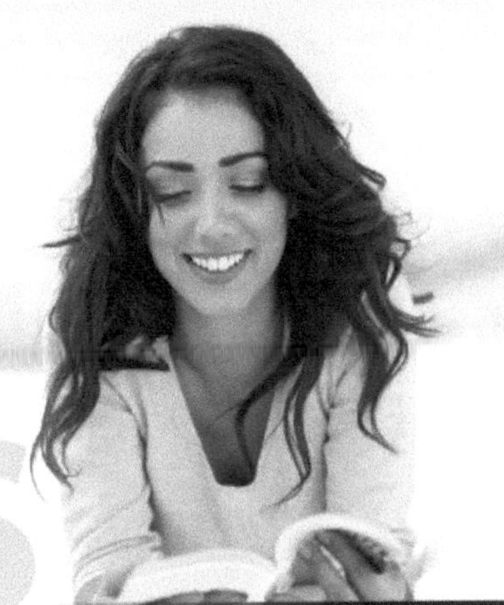

yes

I want morebooks!

Buy your books fast and straightforward online - at one of world's fastest growing online book stores! Environmentally sound due to Print-on-Demand technologies.

Buy your books online at
www.morebooks.shop

Kaufen Sie Ihre Bücher schnell und unkompliziert online – auf einer der am schnellsten wachsenden Buchhandelsplattformen weltweit! Dank Print-On-Demand umwelt- und ressourcenschonend produziert.

Bücher schneller online kaufen
www.morebooks.shop

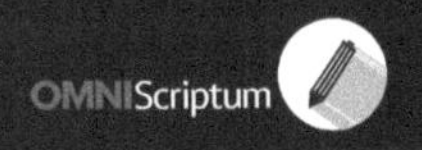

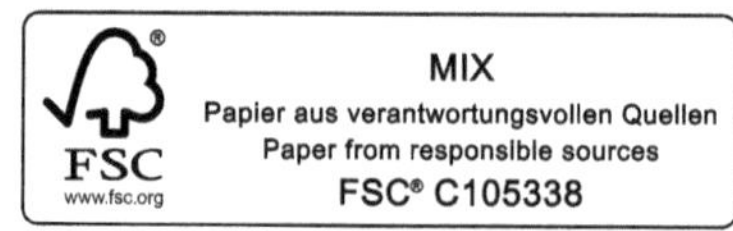

Printed by Books on Demand GmbH, Norderstedt / Germany